I0068189

Dictionary
for End of Life Care

The language of medicine and medications made simple

For non-medical staff, carers and volunteers

Edited by John Ashfield PhD
Foreword by Professor Roderick MacLeod *MNZM*

Dr John Ashfield PhD
© YouCanHelp Publishing 2018
Graphic design: Green Pigeon Graphics – Johanna Evans

IMPORTANT NOTE

The information and ideas in this book are not intended as a substitute for medical or other forms of professional assessment, diagnosis, treatment, or therapy. Some of the information contained here will, over time, be subject to change due to advances in medicines and medications.

All responsibility for editorial matters rests with the author(s). The information and/or self-help resources in this publication are not intended as a substitute for mental health assessment, medical or psychiatric consultation, assessment or treatment.

No part of this document can be reproduced in any way without permission of **YouCanHelp** whose materials are protected under law with a registered trademark.

info@youcanhelp.com.au

ISBN: 978-0-9944664-9-5

Copyright protected you can help

CONTENTS

Foreword

Caring for people near the end of life can be a daunting and frightening task, even for experienced clinicians. For lay people or those with little experience of health care and health care systems it can be similarly worrying. Finding the right time and the right way to introduce concepts of such care has proved difficult for clinicians. When do we adequately try to explain exactly what is going on and how do we do that without using too much jargon?

Palliative care has been identified as a discrete form of clinical practice for over 50 years. It is an approach that improves the quality of life of patients and their families facing the problems associated with life-threatening illness, through the prevention and relief of suffering by means of early identification and impeccable assessment and treatment of pain and other problems, physical, psychosocial and spiritual. As a discipline, it is founded on an interdisciplinary, person-centred model of care delivered by medical, nursing, allied health professionals and volunteers in three settings – home, hospice and hospital. That team must also include the family and informal carers who matter to the person who is dying. Medical people often tend to use words with which they are familiar rather than using the simpler language that is found in everyday use. This dictionary is a way of shining light into dark places where understanding may be poor. By explaining the terms used and outlining the major drugs that may be prescribed it is hoped that some of the uncertainty associated with this phase of life may be minimized. It won't take away all fear, it won't give people more days but it is hoped that it will lighten the load for patient and family alike. I hope it helps.

Prof Rod MacLeod MNZM
Senior Staff Specialist, HammondCare,
Conjoint Professor in Palliative Care, University of Sydney

Introduction

End of life care is a deeply human domain of activity that draws in the many complexities that a life nearing its end unveils, for patients, their families, doctors, nurses and all other carers. Central to this care and always underpinning it are attentive compassion and engaging with the deepest depths of ordinary human experience. Yet, end of life care is also about employing the very best medical knowledge and techniques, and the most efficacious medications appropriate to each individual patient's needs and wishes. This cannot be done without the utility and service of terminology.

This dictionary contains basic medical and pharmaceutical terms in common use in *end of life care* settings such as hospice, palliative care, community care and aged care. The range of entries has been limited to terms and definitions that are particularly useful for non-medical staff, allied health professionals, carers, and volunteers.

Familiarity with some of the language of medicine and medications in end of life care can sometimes aid in better understanding the physical and emotional challenges of terminal illness for patients, and the consequent experience of their families. This knowledge can inform and guide the approach that is taken in counselling and support, and can enhance mutual understanding and better collaboration with doctors and nurses, all bringing potentially better outcomes for those who are the focus of care.

Dr John Ashfield PhD

A

ablation: [ab-lay-shyn]
The surgical removal or amputation of any body part, growth or harmful substance.

abscess: [ab-sess]
A pus-filled cavity surrounded by inflamed tissue.

acute:
Referring to a disease or symptom with rapid onset and marked intensity or severity, subsiding after a short period of time.

acute brain syndrome:
(See **delirium**)

Addison's disease:
A condition caused by partial or complete failure of the adrenal glands. Symptoms include darkening of the pigmentation of the skin and the membranes of the mouth, weakness, weight loss and low blood pressure.

adenocarcinoma: [ad-e-n-o-kar-sin-o-ma]
A cancer within glandular tissue or when cancer cells have a glandular appearance.

adenosarcoma: [ad-e-n-o-sar-ko-ma]
A malignant tumour of glandular and connective tissue.

adhesion: [ad-he-shun]
The union of two surfaces that are normally separate. Abdominal surgery sometimes results in adhesions between loops of bowel from scar tissue.

adjuvant treatment: [ad-ju-vant treatment]
A drug or treatment used in conjunction with another to improve the desired effect. E.g. After surgery, radiotherapy or chemotherapy may be used to improve the chance of disease control.

aetiology: [ee-ti-ol-o-ji]
The study of the cause(s) and origins of disease.

affect: [aff-ect]
A feeling experienced in connection with an emotion or mood.

affective: [aff-ect-ive]
Relates to emotions or moods.

agitation: [aj-it-a-shun]
A mental condition of distress resulting in extreme restlessness.
(see *Pharmaceutical section*)

acquired immune deficiency syndrome: (AIDS)
A condition in which the immune system is damaged due to HIV. This
may result in patients being more vulnerable to unusual infections and
potentially fatal diseases.

alopecia: [al-o-pee-shee-a]
Loss of hair, baldness.

alternative treatments:
Treatments for cancer with no proven physical benefit. Examples
of alternative therapy/treatment: homeopathic, mega-vitamin, and
extreme dietary regimes.

Alzheimer's disease: [al-zime-ers disease]
A progressive, degenerative disorder and the most common form of
dementia. It attacks the brain's nerve cells, or neurons, resulting in loss
of memory, thinking and language skills, and behavioural changes.
It is a disease that leads to death, usually from another illness most
commonly pneumonia. Dementia is the second leading cause of death
in Australia.

ambulatory: [am-bew-late-or-ee]
A word describing a patient who is not confined to bed and is able to
walk. (See *chemotherapy*)

anaemia: [an-ee-me-a]
a) Reduction of the number of red blood cells.
b) Reduction in the amount of haemoglobin in the blood.

anaesthetic: [an-es-thet-ik]
A drug which produces local or general loss of sensibility or sensation.

analgesics: [an-al-gee-ziks]
A drug which acts on the central nervous system to relieve pain.

angiosarcoma: [an-gee-oh-sar-koma]
A rare malignant tumour arising from vascular tissue.

anorexia: [an-or-ex-ia]
Absence of appetite.

anorexia nervosa: [an-o-rex-ia ner-vos-a]
A psychological illness in which an abnormal body image and eating
pattern may result in life threatening weight loss.

antiobiotic: [an-ti-by-otic]
A drug used to prevent the growth of or destroy bacteria.

antibody: [an-ti-body]
A blood protein produced by the body's immune system to defend the body against bacteria or viruses.

anti-coagulant: [an-ti-koh-ag-u-lant]
A substance given to reduce blood clotting. i.e. to 'thin the blood'.

anti-depressant: [an-ti dep-ress-ant]
A medication which can elevate mood. Some types can reduce anxiety and increase coping abilities. (See **Pharmaceutical Section**)

antifungal: [an-ti-fungal]
A substance used to prevent or control fungal infections.

anti-inflammatory:
A substance or medication that counteracts or reduces inflammation. Often produces pain relief.

anxiety: [anks-i-et-ee]
A state of apprehension and fear resulting from the anticipation of a threatening event or situation. The term has also been used to describe the effects of the 'fight or flight' response which is a physiological response to a real or perceived threat.

anxiolytic: [anks-ee-o-lit-ik]
A medication used to treat anxiety episodes.
(See **Pharmaceutical Section**)

aphagia: [a-fay-jee-uh]
Inability to swallow.

aphasia: [a-fay-zee-a]
Inability to speak.

apnoea: [ap-nee-a]
The absence of breathing.

apraxia: [a-prak-see-uh]
Inability to carry out purposeful movements due to a brain lesion, e.g. stroke, brain tumour.

arthralgia: [ar-thral-jee-uh]
Joint pain.

ascites: [as-sigh-teez]
A build up of free fluid in the abdomen (peritoneal cavity) causing distension. Drainage by a large needle (cannula) can effect some relief.

asphyxia: [as-fix-ea]
Obstruction of the nose, mouth or throat causing an inability to breathe.

aspiration: [as-pi-ray-shun]
a) Inadvertent inhalation of a substance into lungs when taking a breath.
b) Drawing off fluid from a body cavity by means of suction.

asthenia: [ass-then-ia]
Loss of strength, weakness, debility.

astrocytoma: [astro-site-oma]
A primary tumour of the brain characterised by slow growth, cyst formation, and slow invasion of surrounding structure. The nature of the tumour may change with time to become more malignant. (see *glioma*).

asymptomatic: [a-simp-to-mat-ik]
Without symptoms.

ataxia: [a-tax-ia]
A condition of impaired physical co-ordination.

atrophy: [at-ro-fee]
A wasting or decrease in size of a normally developed part of the body.

autopsy:
The medical examination of a dead body to determine the cause of death.

axilla: [ax-ill-a]
The armpit.

B

barium enema: [bare-ium en-em-a]
A rectal infusion of barium which allows x-ray examination of the lower intestinal tract. It is used to diagnose tumours, obstructions or other abnormalities.

basal cell carcinoma: [base-al cell kar-sin-o-ma]
Common but least dangerous skin cancer. It grows slowly, but if left untreated a deep ulcer may form and can invade underlying tissue.

benign: [be-nine]
Not malignant.

benign tumour: [be-nine tumour]
Abnormal growth of cells to form a lump or mass, but which does not metastasise to other parts of the body.

benzodiazepines: [ben-so-di-az-a-peenes]
A group of drugs used for their sedative, anxiolytic, muscle relaxant or anti-convulsant effect.

bile:
A liver secretion, stored in the gall bladder which emulsifies fats within the small intestine in preparation for further digestion and absorption.

biliary carcinoma: [billy-ary kar-sin-o-ma]
A relatively rare malignancy in the extrahepatic bile duct, occurring slightly more often in men than in women. It may be associated with progressive jaundice, pruritis, weight loss and, in the later stages, severe pain.

biliousness: [bil-ius-ness]
Term often use to describe nausea, headache and abdominal discomfort.

biochemistry:
The study of the chemistry of living organisms.

biopsy: [by-op-see]
The removal of a small piece of tissue or organ for study to establish a diagnosis. (See **cytology**)

blood count: (See **full blood examination**)

blood type:
Identification of the genetically determined factors on the surface of red blood cells which determine a persons blood group. The main blood types are O, A, B and AB.

bolus: [bole-us]
a) The rounded mass of food prepared by the mouth for swallowing.
b) A single dose of medication usually given all at once, most commonly intravenously.

bone marrow transplant:
A technique where bone marrow cells previously acquired from the patient (when free from malignancy) or from a donor, are infused intravenously. These cells then migrate from the blood stream in to the bone marrow. In some cases the cells are collected (harvested) from the blood (not bone marrow) and the transplant is known as a peripheral blood stem cell transplant.

bone metastases: [bone met-ass-ta-sees]
Secondary cancer growths in the bones. Metastases occur commonly in the axial skeleton (spine, pelvis, skull). The spread occurs through the blood stream. Clinical consequences of bone metastases may be pain, fractures, spinal cord compression and hypercalcaemia. Diagnosis relies on x-rays, bone scans, CAT scans and MRIs.

bowel: [bow-el]
The section of the gastro-intestinal tract between the stomach and anus. The large bowel is comprised of the colon and rectum. The small bowel (or small intestine) is located between the stomach and the colon.

bowel obstruction:
A condition where normal bowel activity and movement is prevented due to adhesion, or tumour pressing against the bowel. It is usually associated with nausea, vomiting, colicky abdominal pain and constipation.

brain metastases: [brain met-ass-ta-sees]
Secondary cancer growth in the brain. 10% of all cancers metastasise to the brain. Clinical features may include headache, vomiting, confusion, epilepsy and stroke.

brain stem:
The lowest part of the brain controlling breathing, swallowing and temperature regulation.

brain tumour:
Tumour growth in the intra-cranial portion of the central nervous system. The most common tumours are brain metastases from a cancer elsewhere. Primary brain tumours are usually gliomas or meningiomas.

brachytherapy: [bra-kee-ther-a-pee]
A form of cancer treatment, especially for prostate cancer, that works by the insertion of radioactive implants directly into the tissue.

bronchial carcinoma: [brong-kial kar-sin-o-ma]
Malignant lung tumour that originates in a bronchus.

bronchodilator: [brong-ko-dye-late-or]
A drug administered to relax the muscle of the bronchial walls to prove ventilation to the lungs.

bronchoscopy: [brong-kos-kop-ee]
An investigation using a bronchoscope to visualise the interior of the trachea or bronchi.

bronchus: [brong-kus]
A large air passage between the trachea and lung tissue.

C

cachexia: [ka-keck-see-uh]
Extreme wasting of the body due to chronic illness, often cancer.

caecum: [see-kum] (See **colon**)

cancer:
A general term used to describe a malignant growth or tumour. Cancerous growths are not self-contained. They can spread to neighbouring tissues and organs via the blood stream or lymph system to form new growth called secondaries or metastases.

candida: [kan-di-da]
A fungus which can cause infection (candidiasis). Occurs in moist areas such as the mouth, vagina and skinfolds. It is also called thrush or monilia and occurs in approximately 70% of patients with advanced cancer.

carcinogen: (kar-sin-o-gen]
An agent which can cause cancer.

carcinoma: (kar-sin-o-ma]
A cancer originating from tissues which comprise the lining of the internal and external surfaces of the body (epithelial tissue). e.g. the skin, bowel, lining of the lungs and other organs.

catheter: [kath-et-er]
A fine tube used to remove or insert fluid into a body cavity. Commonly used to drain the bladder through the urethra.

catheterisation: [kath-et-er-ize-a-shun]
The procedure of inserting a catheter into a body cavity.

computerised axial tomography scan: (CAT Scan)
An x-ray technique producing detailed cross-sectional images of the body. Assists in the identification of tumour masses and accumulations of fluid. Sometimes called CT scan.

central nervous system: (CNS)
Comprises cerebral hemispheres, cerebellum, brain stem and spinal cord.

cervical spine: [ser-vike-al spine]
The bones of the neck. There are usually seven bones forming the cervical vertebra.

cervix: [sir-vix]
The neck of the uterus (womb) which projects into the vagina.

chemotherapy: [keem-o-therapy]
Treatment of disease by the administration of drugs. There are different types of chemotherapy used to prevent or slow down the growth of cells at different stages of cell division. Drugs can be administered by mouth, by intravenous injection or occasionally by infusion into a particular organ e.g. liver. Ambulatory chemotherapy refers to a continuous infusion of chemotherapy delivered over several days as the patient continues their normal activities.

Cheyne-Stokes respiration:
An abnormal pattern of breathing characterised by alternating periods of apnoea and deep, rapid breathing. This may signify approaching death.

chromosomes: [kro-mo-somes]
Structures located in the nucleus of a cell which contain all the information for cell growth and function. Chromosomes contain thousands of genes. Cancer cell abnormalities can sometimes be detected in chromosomes.

chronic: [kro-nic]
Of long duration. (The opposite of acute.)

chronic obstructive airways disease (COAD):
(See **chronic obstructive pulmonary disease** (COPD))

chronic obstructive pulmonary disease (COPD):
A progressive and irreversible disease of the lung characterised by diminished inspiratory and expiratory capacity.

cirrhosis: [si-ro-sis]
A degenerative condition of the liver. Causes include alcohol, toxins, infections and severe malnutrition.

clinical trial:
Scientific study involving patients, to determine the effectiveness of a new treatment or to compare treatments. Clinical trials are only conducted after tests have established that the new treatment is unlikely to be detrimental to the patient.

coccyx: [kok-siks]
The bone at the base of the spinal column, where four vertebrae are fused to form a small triangle.

cognitive: [cog-nit-iv]
Referring to mental processes, (thinking and reasoning powers).

colectomy: [ko-lect-om-ee]
Surgical excision of the colon as a treatment for cancer and some benign inflammatory diseases of the bowel.

colitis: [ko-lie-tis]
Inflammation of the colon.

colon: [ko-lon]
The large intestine. The section of the bowel from the small intestine to the rectum. The colon is usually described in sections:
a) caecum (cul-de-sac at the beginning of the large intestine)
b) ascending colon (right hemi-colon)
c) transverse colon
d) descending colon (left hemi-colon)
e) sigmoid colon (loop of colon between the descending colon and the rectum.)

colonic cancer: [ko-lon-ik kan-ser] (See **colorectal cancer**).

colonoscope: [ko-lon-os-kope]
A fibre-optic instrument inserted through the anus to allow a visual examination of the interior of the large intestine (colon).

colonoscopy: [kol-on-os-kopy]
The visual examination of the large intestine using a colonoscope.

colorectal: [kol-o-rek-tal] (See *bowel*)

colorectal cancer: [kol-or-rectal kan-ser]
A malignant neoplastic disease of the large intestine. Warning signs may be a change in bowel habit, and the passing of blood. Malignant tumours of the large bowel usually occur after the age of 50 and are slightly more frequent in women than men. There may be hereditary factors.

colostomy: [kol-los-toh-mee]
A surgical procedure which creates a temporary or permanent opening through the abdominal wall into the colon, permitting the elimination of faeces into a colostomy bag.

colposcopy: [kol-pos-ko-pee]
The visual examination of the vagina and uterine cervix with a magnifying instrument to detect benign and malignant changes and to enable selective biopsy. This can aid early detection of pre-cancerous changes.

coma:
A state of unconsciousness when the patient cannot be roused.

comatose: [kome-uh-tose]
The state of coma.

complementary therapies:
Supportive therapies which are used alongside orthodox medical care to improve the quality of a patient's life.

compression fracture:
A fracture of bone that is the result of two bone surfaces having been forced towards each other.

confusion:
When consciousness is clouded, the capacity to think is disrupted, perception is dulled and response is less acute.

congestive cardiac failure:
A condition characterised by circulatory congestion caused by heart disorders.

constipation:
Accumulation of hardened faces which is difficult to evacuate. This is a frequent and sometimes severe problem for terminally ill patients. It may be due to drugs, dehydration, low fibre diet, depression, immobility, inadequate physical activity, tumour obstruction of the bowel and hypercalcaemia. (See *faecal impaction*)

convulsion:
A spasmodic or prolonged involuntary series of contractions of a group of muscles due to cerebral irritation or dysfunction. Also called a seizure or fit.

cordotomy: [kor-dot-om-y]
Surgical procedure on spinal cord, dividing specific nerve pathways to relieve intractable pain.

cranial: [cray-nee-al]
Of or relating to the cranium.

cranium: [cray-nee-um]
The part of the skull that encloses and protects the brain.

cure:
Total abolition of a particular disease in a patient.

cutaneous: [kute-ane-eus]
Pertaining to the skin.

cyanosis: [sigh-an-o-sis]
Bluish appearance of the skin due to imperfect oxygenation of blood. The condition can be an indication of circulatory failure.

cyst: [sist]
A cavity or sac containing liquid or semi-solid matter.

cystoscopy: [sis-toss-ko-pee]
Visual examination of the bladder, through the urethra using a cystoscope. A cystoscopy may also be used for removal of small growth and to collect tissue for a biopsy.

cytology: [sigh-tol-o-jee]
The science of the microscopic study of the cells of the body. An aid to early diagnosis of malignant disease. Cells can only be collected by a fine needle from body tissues or fluids (FNA or fine needle aspirate) or from smears e.g. cervical, or from body secretions e.g. sputum or urine.

cytotoxic: [sigh-toh-tox-ik]
Refers to an agent that damages or inhibits the growth of cells. (See **chemotherapy**)

D

death rate:
The number of deaths in a set period and given number of population. Sometimes called mortality rate.

death rattle:
A gurgling sound sometimes heard in a dying person's throat when secretions collect in the trachea and move up and down with respiration. Often heard as a patient nears death.

debulking:
Generally refers to the surgical excision and removal of a significant proportion of a tumour, for palliative effect.

decubitus ulcer: [de-ku-bi-tus ulcer]
Commonly called 'pressure sores', decubitus ulcers appear in the skin over areas of bony prominence, and are most frequent in immobilised patients.

degenerative disease:
Any disease that is characterised by a deterioration of tissue structure or function.

dehydration:
An excessive loss of water from the body tissues. Signs can include thirst, loss of skin elasticity and sunken eyes.

delirium: [de-lear-e-um]
A state of confusion usually with a reduced level of consciousness due to an acute organic mental disorder. Often characterised by disorientation, fear, restlessness, anxiety, delusions and frequently hallucinations.

dementia: [de-men-sha]
Describes a collection of symptoms that are caused by organic brain disease. It is not one specific disease. Dementia may adversely affect thinking, memory, personality, and behaviour. It can cause confusion, disorientation, and impairment of judgment. It often interferes with a person's capacity to perform everyday tasks. It is the second leading cause of death in Australia (see **Alzheimer's disease** the most common form of dementia).

depression:
May be one of several disorders:
a) Disruptive mood dysregulation disorder
b) Major depressive disorder (including major depressive episode)
c) Persistent depressive disorder (dysthymia)
d) Premenstrual dysphoric disorder
e) Substance/medication-induced depressive disorder
f) Depressive disorder due to another medical condition
g) Other specified depressive disorder
h) Unspecified depressive disorder.

The characteristics all these forms of depression have in common are: the presence of a sad, empty, or irritable mood, accompanied by changes in bodily and mental functioning that significantly affect a person's capacity to function. What makes these kinds of depression different are issues of duration, timing, or presumed cause or reason for the condition.

Though bereavement-related grief and major depressive disorder share some features in common, they are distinct and distinguishable conditions. And, though bereavement is a common precipitant of clinical depression, recognising major depressive disorder in the context of recent bereavement requires careful clinical assessment and judgment, and by no means implies that antidepressant treatment is warranted.

diagnosis:
The process of identifying a disease. Diagnosis involves taking a history by questioning and examining the patient, and if necessary performing laboratory and X-ray investigations. Differential diagnosis is the process of considering all the possible explanations for a particular set of symptoms or signs.

diaphragm: [dye-uh-fram]
The muscular partition which separates the chest from the abdomen. It is the chief muscle of respiration.

diarrhoea: [dye-uh-rea]
Frequent discharge of abnormally liquid faces.

diathermy: [dye-uh-thur-mee]
An electric current used during surgical operations to stop bleeding or to destroy abnormal tissue.

differentiated cells:
Cells which are specialised and have function which differentiate them from other cells. Malignant cells can be graded according to their degree of differentiation. Usually differentiated tumours carry the worst prognosis.

disseminated cancer: [dis-sem-i-nat-ed cancer]
Cancer which is widely scattered and dispersed (metastasised) throughout the body.

dissociative [diss-o-soh-shee-a-tive]
Relating to a state of consciousness or mental process where a person experiences some degree of detachment (from mild to severe) from their thoughts, feelings, memories or sense of identity. This involves a degree of detachment from reality, rather than a loss of reality as in psychosis.

distended:
A term commonly used to describe abdominal swelling from pressure inside.

diuresis: [dye-you-re-sis]
Increased or excessive production of urine.

diuretic: [dye-you-ret-ik]
A drug or other substance which promotes the production and flow of urine. Diuretics reduce the volume of extracellular fluid and assist in the treatment of oedema and a range of disorders including hypertension and congestive heart failure.

dysarthria: [dis-arth-ree-a]
Impairment of articulation of speech.

dyspepsia: [dis-pep-see-uh]
Flatulence, nausea and at times vomiting. Anxiety and tension can aggravate the symptoms.

dysphagia: [dis-fay-jee-uh]
Difficulty in swallowing.

dysphasia: [dis-fay-zee-uh]
Difficulty in speaking or understanding language due to a brain lesion.

dysplasia: [dis-play-zee-uh]
Tissue which develops abnormally but is not malignant. Occasionally it may progress to malignancy.

dyspnoea: [disp-nee-ah]
Laboured and difficult breathing, shortness of breath.

dystonia: [dis-toe-nee-ah]
Impairment of normal muscle tone, characterised by muscle spasm or flaccidity (loose, limp, soft muscle).

dysuria: [dis-u-ree-a]
Pain or discomfort when passing urine.

E

effleurage: [ef-lu-rahzh]
A massage technique which facilitate dispersal of oedema.

effusion: [e-fu-shun]
A collection of blood or fluid in a body cavity.

electrolyte: [elec-tro-lite]
Refers to the salts in the blood stream or body. A normal balance of electrolytes in the body is essential to health.

emaciation: [em-ace-i-a-shun]
A wasting of body tissue caused by disease or lack of nutrition.

embolism: [em-bol-ism]
A condition in which a blood clot, fat or air moves through the circulatory system and obstructs blood vessels, e.g. Pulmonary embolism – blood clot in the lungs.

emesis: [em-a-sis]
The act of vomiting.

emphysema: [em-fi-see-mah]
A condition whereby the air sacs of the lungs are destroyed, interfering with the effective surface area in the lungs for exchange of gases. Severe cases may exhibit difficulty in breathing.

encephalitis: [en-sef-a-lite-is or en-sef-a-lite-is]
Inflammation of the brain and its coverings (the meninges).

encephalomyelitis: [en-kef-al-oh-mya-lite-is or en-sef-al-oh-mya-lite-is)
Inflammation of the brain and spinal cord.

encephalopathy: en-kef-al-op-athy or en-sef-al-op-athy]
Any disease of the brain, affecting the structure or function of tissues of the brain.

endocrine: [en-doh-kreen]
Relating to or denoting glands which secrete hormones or other products directly into the blood.

endocrinologist: [en-doh-kri-nol-o-jist]
A doctor specialising in the diagnosis and treatment of the diseases of endocrine glands.

endometrial: [en-doh-met-ri-al]
Pertaining to the lining of the uterus.

endoscope: [en-doh-skope]
An optical instrument used to illuminate and observe the interior of a body cavity.

endoscopy: [en-dos-ko-pee]
The use of an endoscope to visualise the interior of a body cavity or organ. Usually refers to the oesophagus or stomach.

enuresis: [en-u-re-sis]
The involuntary passing or urine at night.

epidemiology: [ep-i-dee-me-il-o-jee]
The study of the distribution and determinants of diseases.

epidural: [ep-i-dure-al]
An epidural anaesthetic, used to produce loss of sensation below the waist.

epidural catheter: [ep-i-dure-al kath-et-er]
A fine tube inserted into the epidural space of the spinal column through which anaesthetic or other medication is administered, e.g. analgesics.

epithelium: [ep-i-theel-eum]
The surface cells which constitute the skin or lining tissue.

erythrocytes: [e-rith-row-sites]
Red blood cells which are produced in the bone marrow.

Ewing's sarcoma: [u-ings sar-koma]
A malignant tumour which develops from bone marrow in the shaft of long bones or the pelvis. Usually occurs in young people.

excision: [ek-sizh-shun]
The cutting of tissue from the body.

F

faecal impaction: [fee-kal impaction]
The condition that is a result of a collection of hardened faeces in the rectum, or sigmoid. Liquid faces may leak around the impaction and appear as diarrhoea – spurious diarrhoea.

familial polyposis: [familial pol-ip-o-sis]
A condition characterised by the development of polyps in the colon and rectum. The tendency is inherited and the potential for malignancy is high.

fistula: [fis-tu-lah]
An abnormal opening between two internal organs or between an internal organ and the surface of the skin.

full blood examination (FBE):
A laboratory test to assess red and white blood cells and platelet numbers in the blood. (Also known as complete blood examination – CBE or full blood count – FBC).

fungal infection:
An inflammatory condition caused by a fungal organism.

fungating tumour:
A visible tumour that has the appearance of a fungus like mass.

fungus:
A simple plant form. Some fungi may cause infections in humans.

G

gall bladder:
A pear shaped sac located below the liver. It is a reservoir for bile. The gall bladder aids in the digestion of fats by releasing bile into the small intestine.

gall bladder cancer:
A malignant tumour of the gall bladder which rarely occurs before the age of 40 years. It is characterised by nausea, anorexia, vomiting, weight loss, pain in the upper abdomen and jaundice.

gastric carcinoma:
Malignant tumour of the stomach. The incidence is higher in men than in women and peaks in the 50 – 59 year old age group.

gastrointestinal tract: [gas-tro-in-tes-tie-nal tract]
The alimentary tract: pertains to the mouth, oesophagus, stomach, bowel and anus.

gerontology: [jer-on-tol-o-jee]
The study of the ageing process.

glioma: [gli-o-mah]
A tumour composed of cells and fibres representative of the special supporting tissues of the central nervous systems. Gliomas occur in the brain and spinal cord. The most malignant form is known as gliobastoma multiforme. (See **brain tumour**.)

glossectomy:
Surgical excision of the tongue.

glucose:
A simple sugar which can be ingested, or produced by digestion, and which is readily absorbed into the blood from the intestines. It is a primary source of energy for the body. The examination of glucose levels in the blood remains an important diagnostic test in diabetes and other disorders.

gray:
Unit of radiation therapy. One Gray (Gy) equals 100 rad.

gynaecologist: [guy-na-kol-o-jist]
A doctor specialising in the diseases unique to female genital tract.

H

haematemesis: [hee-muh-tem-a-sis]
The vomiting of blood.

haematologist: [hee-muh-tol-o-jist]
A doctor who specialises in dealing with the nature, function and diseases of the blood.

haematology: [hee-muh-tol-o-jee]
The study of the blood and blood-producing organs.

haematoma: [hee-muh-toh-mah]
A swelling containing blood.

haematuria: [hee-muh-ture-eah]
The presence of blood in the urine.

haemoglobin: [hee-muh-globe-in]
The substance which gives red blood cells their colour, and transports oxygen from the lungs to the cells.

haemoptysis: [hee-mop-ti-sis]
Coughing of blood.

haemorrhage: [hem-o-rij]
Bleeding, may be internal or external.

halitosis: [hal-it-o-sis]
Offensive smelling breath.

hallucination: [hah-lu-si-na-shun]
False perception. May be visual, auditory, tactile, gustatory (taste) or olfactory (smell).

hallucinogen: [hal-lu-si-no-jen]
A drug which induces hallucinations.

hemi-colectomy:
Surgical excision of one of the portions of the colon.

hepatic: [hep-at-ik]
Relating to the liver.

hepatomegaly: [hep-ah-to-meg-ah-lee]
An abnormal enlargement of the liver, usually indicative of liver disease.

herpes simplex: [her-peez sim-plex] or cold sores:
An infection caused by herpes simplex virus (HSV), which affects the skin and nervous system. It becomes evident through small, sometimes painful, fluid filled blisters on the skin and mucous membranes.
HSV 1 (oral herpes) tends to manifest in the facial area – especially around the mouth and nose.
HSV 2 (genital herpes) is usually limited to the genital region.
Herpes viruses are extremely contagious.

histology: [hist-ol-o-jee]
The study of the microscopic structure, composition and function of body tissues.

human immunodeficiency virus: (HIV)
A human retrovirus that is blood borne, usually transmitted sexually or by exchange of body fluids or blood, e.g. sharing needles in intravenous drug users. This causes an infection which can lead to AIDS and other related diseases.

Hodgkin's disease:
A malignant disorder which causes progressive enlargement of lymphoid tissue. Treatment is radiotherapy and cytotoxic drugs. Long term remissions are achievable in more than 50% of patients.

holistic care:
Care pertaining to the whole person; care that seeks to address physical, psychological, social, and spiritual needs.

hormone:
A chemical substance produced by one organ, which may then be transported by the blood to other organs or tissues where it acts to modify their structure or function.

hormone receptors:
On the surface of some cancer cells, there may be receptors which indicate that the cancer may be responsive to hormone treatment.

hormone therapy:
A cancer treatment that is used to suppress the production of or inhibit the effects of a hormone (such as estrogen or testosterone), most commonly to treat breast or prostate cancer. Hormone therapy is also called hormonal therapy, hormone treatment, or endocrine therapy.

hospice:
'A hospice is a team or community concerned with enhancing the quality of remaining life for a patient and family struggling with mortal illness.' (Cicely Saunders). Alternatively: the medical and nursing facility in which the hospice care is carried out.

hospice care:
The coordinated provision of medical, emotional and spiritual support for dying people and their families. Hospice care usually involves provision of care in a patient's home or in a home like setting. It also involves the support of bereaved families. Modern hospice (palliative) care can also provide pain or symptom management prior to the terminal phase of the illness. (See **terminal**)

hypercalcaemia: [hy-per-kal-see-mee-ah]
Condition where there is a high level of calcium in the blood. If the condition is untreated it may lead to anorexia, confusion, drowsiness, coma and ultimately death.

hyperglycaemia: [hy-po-gly-see-mee-ah]
An excess of glucose in the blood.

hypocalcaemia: [hy-po-kal-see-mee-uh]
Diminished calcium in the blood.

hypodermoclysis: [hy-po-der-mok-ly-sis]
The infusion of a solution into the subcutaneous (below the skin) tissue, to provide a patient with a continuous quantity of fluid, to compensate for inadequate intake or loss of water and salt.

hypoglycaemia: [hy-per-gly-see-mee-ah-
An abnormally low level of glucose in the blood.

hypoxia: [hy-pok-see-ah]
A broad term meaning diminished availability of oxygen to the body tissues. Hypoxia may lead to mental confusion.

hysterectomy: [hiss-ter-ek-toh-mee]
Removal of the uterus.

I

ileal conduit: [ill-e-al kon-duit]
A new bladder is made from a loop of small bowel (ileum) and drained into a ileostomy bag.

ileostomy [ill-e-os-toe-mee]
A surgical operation in which a damaged part is removed from the ileum (the third portion of the small intestine) and the cut end diverted to an artificial opening in the abdominal wall.

ileus: [ill-e-us]
An obstruction of the intestine. The term is generally used when the obstruction is due to bowel immobility rather than mechanical blockage.

immunology:
The study of the body's defence mechanisms and immunity.

immunosuppression: [im-mune-o-sup-presh-on]
Inhibited functioning of the immune system. This results in reduction if the body's natural defences, which may further result in infections and cancers of the skin and lymphoid tissue. Immunosuppression may be a side effect of radiotherapy and chemotherapy.

immunotherapy: [im-mune-o therapy]
A treatment that uses certain parts of a person's immune system to fight diseases such as cancer.

impalpable: [im-palp-able]
Unable to be felt by manual examination.

incidence:
The number of new cases of disease occurring in a defined population over a specific period of time.

incontinence: [in-kon-tin-ence]
The inability to control natural excretory functions.

Infarct: [in-far-kt]
Necrosis of part of the or the whole of an organ caused by the blockage of a blood vessel, usually due to an embolus (blood clot, fat, air, amniotic fluid or a foreign body).

infarction: [in-fark-shun]
Necrosis following the interruption of blood supply to any part or all of an organ.
myocardial – infarction of the heart muscle following coronary thrombosis.
pulmonary – infraction of part of the lung resulting from obstruction in the pulmonary artery.

inflammation:
The reaction of tissue to injury. The injury may result from infections, or physical or chemical damage, or immune reactions.

infusion:
The injections of a fluid (drug, nutrient or electrolyte) directly into a vein or subcutaneously (under the skin) by pump or gravity flow.

infusion pump:
Equipment designed to administer a set amount of a drug or fluid over a set period of time.

insomnia:
Inability to sleep or remain asleep. May be caused by physical and psychological factors.

intestinal obstruction: (See **bowel obstruction**)

intractable:
Unable to be relieved, restrained or cured.

intrathecal: [in-tra-thee-kal]
Within the membranes covering the spinal cord.

intrathecal catheter:
A fine tube which is inserted next to the spinal cord through which anaesthetic and/or analgesic medication is administered continuously or intermittently.

intravenous injection (I.V.)
Injection of medication or fluid into a vein.

irrigation:
Procedure of washing out a cavity or wound with a stream of water, saline or other solution.

J

jaundice: [jawn-dis]
A yellow discolouration of the skin due to the presence of bile pigment in the blood. May be associated with dark urine, pale faeces and often causes itching.

K

Kaposi's sarcoma: [Kap-o-si's sar-ko-ma]
A malignancy which begins as soft, brownish or purple papules (raised lumps) on the skin and slowly spreads metastasising to the lymph nodes and internal organs.

L

labile: [lay-bile]
Unstable, subject to tendency to change.

laparoscopy: [lap-ar-os-ko-pee]
A procedure whereby an instrument is introduced through a small hole in the abdominal wall to examine the internal organs.

laparotomy: [lap-a-rot-o-mee]
An operation to open the abdominal wall so that internal organs can be visually examined.

laryngectomy: [la-rin-ject-o-mee]
Partial or total removal of the larynx as a treatment for cancer of the larynx.

larynx: [la-rinks]
The hollow organ forming part of the air passage to the lungs, containing the vocal cords and producing the sound heard in speech.

laser surgery:
Surgery using lasers can divide adhesions, destroy or fix tissue into place. It is a valuable procedure when conventional surgery is unable to access particular areas of the body.

leiomyosarcoma: [lye-o-my-osar-ko-ma]
A malignant tumour consisting of smooth muscle cells.

lesion:
A general term for a wound, injury or other pathological change in body tissue.

lethargy:
An abnormal lack of energy exhibited by dullness, sluggishness or indifference.

leucocyte: [loo-ko-site]
A white blood cell.

leucopoenia: [loo-ko-peen-ia]
A reduced number of white blood cells to below 3,000 per cubic millimetre of whole blood. Usual number of white blood cells is between 4,000 and 11,000 per cubic millimetre. (see **neutropenia**)

leukaemia: [loo-key-me-a]
Malignant disease of the blood forming tissues, bone marrow and blood forming organs. Leukaemias may occur is several different forms and may be described by the rate of their progression (acute or chronic) and according to the type of white blood cells which are affected. (e.g. lymphoid or myeloid)

leukoplakia: [loo-ko-play-kee-a]
A precancerous, slowly developing change in a mucous membrane, manifesting in thickened white patches, occurring on the lips, tongue or gums, or on the penis or vulva. Leukoplakia, if not treated, has a tendency to become malignant.

liposarcoma: [lip-o-sar-ko-ma]
A malignant tumour of the fat cells.

liver:
A large organ situated in the upper right part of the abdomen.
Its main functions are:
a) the secretion of bile
b) purification of the blood
c) regulation of metabolic processes.

liver cancer:
Not a common primary cancer. Usually represents a metastasis from another site, e.g. bowel, bladder or breast.

lobectomy: [lo-bek-toh-mee]
Surgical removal of a lobe of the lung or the liver usually due to the presence of a malignant tumour.

lumbar spine:
The portion of the spine in the small of the back (between the thorax and the pelvis).

lumpectomy: [lum-pek-toh-mee]
An operation involving the removal of a tumour without removing large amounts of surrounding tissue or adjacent lymph glands.
e.g. breast lumpectomy – the removal of a breast lump or cancer with preservation of the breast.

lung cancer:
A pulmonary malignancy commonly attributed to smoking. Lung cancers are classified according to the type of cell involved. Cancer most often will develop in scarred or diseased lungs, and can be quite advanced before being detected. The lungs are also a common site for metastatic cancer.

lungs:
A pair of conical organs in the respiratory system. In the lungs, oxygen is absorbed from the inspired air and carbon dioxide is exhaled.

lymph: [limf]
A clear fluid from the blood which has passed through the capillary walls to supply nutrients to tissue cells. Lymph collects into lymph vessels through which it is ultimately returned to the blood.
Lymphadenopathy: [limf-ad-en-op-a-thee]
Enlargement of the lymph nodes.

lymphatic system: [limf-at-ik system]
Complex circulatory network of vessels, valves, ducts, nodes and organs that carries lymph.

lymph nodes: (also called lymph glands)
Small oval shaped structures situated along the course of lymph vessels. Most of the lymph nodes are clustered in the neck, axilla and the groins. Also occur deep in the abdomen (retroperitoneal nodes) and chest (mediastinal nodes). Cancer cells from a primary tumour can spread through the lymphatic system to other parts of the body.

lymphoblast: [limf-o-blast]
A cell that is immature but could develop into a lymphocyte.

lymphocyte: [limf-oh-cite]
A white blood cell formed in the lymphoid tissue. These cells are involved in immune reactions.

lymphoedema: [limf-oh-deem-a]
A subcutaneous accumulation of lymph resulting from damaged or blocked lymphatic vessels.

lymphogram: [limf-oh-gram]
An X-ray examination of lymph glands and lymph vessels after the injection of a contrast medium (dye).

lymphoid tissue: [limf-oid tissue]
Tissue in which the lymphocytes are produced: the lymph glands, bone marrow and spleen. This tissue is crucial to a patient's ability to fight infections.

lymphoma: [limf-o-mah]
A term referring to any malignant condition which has its origin in the lymphoid tissue. These diseases can generally be classified into two categories: either Hogkins or non-Hodgkins lymphomas.

M

malabsorption:
Impairment of normal absorption of nutrients.

malaise:
A vague feeling of general discomfort and weakness which often marks the onset of disease.

malignant tumour:
A tumour which invades surrounding tissue and/or spreads (metastasises) to distant sites where new tumours may develop.

mammography: [mam-og-raff-ee]
Radiographic examination of the soft tissues of the breast which can identify abnormal growths. It may be possible to detect cancer before a tumour can be felt.

mammoplasty:
Reshaping or reconstruction of the breasts by a plastic surgeon.

manual removal:
The removal of faeces from the rectum by hand (usually with one finger).

marrow:
The soft tissue contained in the middle of the long bones. It is comprised of myeloid tissue which is vital in the production and maturation of red blood cells.

mastectomy: [mas-teek-toh-mee]
The amputation of the breast. Radical mastectomy refers to the removal of breast tissue, axillary lymph glands and the pectoral muscle. If both breast are removed the procedure is referred to as a bilateral mastectomy.

mediastinum: [mee-di-a-stine-um]
The central section of the chest between the lungs extending from the sternum to the vertebral column. It contains the heart and large blood vessels, trachea, oesophagus and lymph nodes.

malaena: [meh-lee-na]
The passage of altered blood with the bowel motion – usually appears black and sticky.

melanoma: [mel-an-o-ma]
A malignant tumour which is usually pigmented and may originate anywhere on the skin or in mucous membranes. It can metastasise widely. Prognosis is determined according to the type of melanoma, its dimensions, location, age and health of the patient. Melanoma may develop in pre-existing moles or freckles or sun-damaged skin.

meningioma: [men-in-je-o-mah]
A tumour of the membranes enveloping the brain and spinal cord. Often slow growing, usually vascular. They usually occur in adults.

meningitis: [men-in-jite-is]
Inflammation of the membranes (meninges) that cover the brain and spinal cord.

mesothelioma: [meez-o-theel-io-ma]
A rare but rapidly growing tumour of the membrane covering the lung (pleura). It is associated with exposure to unstable asbestos usually 15-20 years prior to diagnosis. More rarely arises from the lining of the peritoneal cavity.

metabolism:
The physical and chemical processes concerned with the conversion of nutrients into energy.

metaplasia: [met-a-play-ze-ah]
A condition in which normal tissue cell structure converts to an abnormal form in response to chronic stress or injury. This condition may indicate a malignant change.

metastases: [met-as-ta-sees]
Plural of metastasis.

metastasis: [met-as-ta-sis]
A tumour which is the result of cancer cells moving from a primary site via the blood stream or lymphatic channels.

metastasise: [me-tas-tah-size]
The process by which tumour cells are spread to distant parts of the body via blood vessels and lymphatic channels. Metastasising is one of the characteristics of cancer. These new growth are called secondaries or metastases.

micturition: [mik-ture-i-shun]
The act of passing urine.

monoclonal antibodies: [mon-o-clo-nol anti-bod-ees]
Man-made antibodies designed to specifically target and lock onto a certain antigen (substance that can be recognised by the immune system), such as one found on cancer cells. Monoclonal antibodies are used to treat many diseases including some forms of cancer.

morbidity:
The statistical measurement of the incidence of illness, sickness or disability.

moribund:
A state of being near death, listless and without energy.

mortality:
The number of deaths in proportion to the population: The statistical measurement of the incidence of deaths.

Motor neurone disease:
A chronic progressive disease affecting the nerve cells that transmit impulses to muscular or glandular tissue, resulting in functional impairment.

mucus: [mew-kus]
The slippery viscous secretion of mucous glands and membranes containing mucin, that lubricates body surfaces protecting them from friction or erosion.

multiple myeloma: [multiple my-e-lo-ma] (See *myeloma*)

multiple sclerosis: (M.S.): [multiple skler-ro-sis]
A disease of the nervous system characterised by areas of damage (plaques) occurring randomly in the brain and spinal cord, resulting in interference with the nerves in those areas, and giving rise to a broad range of symptoms. In advanced disease, emotional stability (lability), impairment of physical coordination, reflexes, and urination, are common.

muscular dystrophy:
A group of genetically transmitted muscular diseases that are progressively crippling as muscles weaken and eventually atrophy.

mutation: [mew-t-shun]
Abnormal change in genetic makeup of a cell, either spontaneously or by induction (e.g. radiation).

myalgia: [my-al-je-ah]
Muscle pain.

myasthenia: [my-ass-theen-ee-a]
A condition characterised by muscle debility or weakness.

myeloblast: [my-lo-blast]
An immature cell in the bone marrow which will eventually mature into granular leucocytes (white blood cell). Myeloblasts are the malignant white blood cells in myeloblastic leukaemia.

myeloid: [my-e-loid]
Pertaining to, derived from, or resembling bone marrow.

myeloma: [my-e-lo-ma]
A tumour composed of cells normally found in the bone marrow. It may develop at more than one site and cause destruction of the bone.

myopathy: [my-op-athee]
A disease of skeletal muscle, characterised by weakness and wasting.

myosarcoma: [my-o-sar-koma]
A malignant tumour of the muscle.

N

narcosis: [nar-ko-sis]
a) A state of sleep.
b) An unconscious state produced by a narcotic drug.

narcotic: [nar-kot-ik]
A substance that produces insensibility or sleep. A narcotic analgesic usually refers to a drug derived from opium (such as morphine) or produced synthetically for the treatment of pain.

nausea: [naw-ze-ah]
A sensation of sickness or an inclination to vomit. Nausea and vomiting occur in approximately 60% of cancer patients at some stage of the disease.

necrosis: [nek-ro-sis]
Death of a section of tissue or organ which occurs in response to disease or injury.

neoplasm: [neo-plasm]
An abnormal new growth. The growth may be benign or malignant.
(See **tumour**)

nephroblastoma: [nef-ro-blass-to-ma] (See: **Wilms' tumour**)

nephroma: [nef-ro-ma]
A tumour of the kidney.

neuralgia: [nu-ral-je-ah]
Severe stabbing pain originating from a disorder or disease affecting
the nervous system.

neurogenic: [nu-ro-jen-ik]
Originating in the nervous system.

neuroleptic: [nu-ro-lep-tik]
A drug which reduces motor activity, anxiety and induces indifference
to the surroundings.

neurology: [nu-rol-o-gee]
The field of medicine which studies the nervous system.

neuroma: [nu-roma]
A benign tumour which consists of nervous tissue.

neuropathic: [nu-ro-path-ik]
Refers to a disease process affecting the nerves.

neutropenia: [nu-tro-pee-nia]
A reduction in the number of white blood cells particularly involved in
fighting bacterial infection. A common side effect of chemotherapy.

nightmare:
A dream experienced as fearful, intense and distressing, occurring
during rapid eye movement sleep, and which usually awakens the
sleeper.

night terror:
Repeated and abrupt awakening from sleep with an experience of
panic, anxiety, disorientation and often a scream, with no memory
about the vent. May be related to fatigue, stress, or the use of tricyclic
antidepressants or neuroleptic medications.

node:
A small round shaped protuberance or swelling which could be normal
or abnormal.

non-Hodgkin's lymphoma: [non-Hodgkins limf-oh-mah]
Any kind of malignant lymphoma except Hodgkin's disease.

non-medical treatments:
A large range of alternative and complementary therapies. These may include herbal remedies, special diets, imagery, lifestyle modifications, meditation, spiritual healing, secret remedies and medicines.

O

oat cell carcinoma: (See **Small Cell Carcinoma**)

oedema: [uh-dee-muh]
Excessive fluid accumulation in body tissues. Pressing a finger upon the affected tissue area will usually produce a depression (pit), then slowly the original contour is regained.

oesophageal cancer: [e-sof-ah-jee-al cancer]
A malignant tumour of the oesophagus, occurring more frequently in men than in women, and which may spread locally or may metastasise to lymph nodes, lungs and liver. It may obstruct swallowing.

oesophageal speech: [e-so-ah-jee-al speech]
Speaking by vibrating the air in the oesophagus. This method may be used by a patient who has had a laryngectomy (the voice box removed).

oesphagitis: [e-so-a-jy-tis]
Inflammation of the oesophagus.

oesophagus: [e-sof-ah-gus]
The hollow muscular tube extending from the throat to the stomach.

oncologist: [on-kol-o-jist]
A doctor who specialises in the study, prevention, diagnosis, treatment, and management of cancer.

opioid: [oh-pee-oid] (also known as opiate)
Any drug derived from opium or other semi synthetic or synthetic drug with opium-like activity, e.g. morphine, oxycodone.

organic:
Pertaining to the internal organs of the body. Implies a physical rather than psychological disease.

oestrogenic sarcoma: [osti-o-jen-ik sar-koma]
A malignant bone tumour, commonly affecting young adults.

osteolytic: [ost-e-o-lit-ik]
The dissolution of the bone.

osteoma: [os-tee-oh-mah]
A tumour composed of bone.

ostomy: [os-toh-mee]
A surgical procedure where an artificial opening is made. Each procedure is named after the anatomic location of the opening (e.g. colostomy or cystostomy). (See **stoma**)

ovarian cancer:
A malignant neoplastic disease of the ovary occurring most frequently in women between the ages of 40 and 60 and occasionally in young adolescents.

ovary:
One of a pair of female glandular organs which produce ova (eggs).

P

paediatrics: [pee-dee-at-triks]
The branch of medicine specialising in children and their diseases.

palliative: [pall-ee-ah-tiv]
Originally from the Latin meaning to 'cover' or 'cloak'.
Palliative care is an approach that improves the quality of life of patients and their families facing the problem associated with life-threatening illness, through the prevention and relief of suffering by means of early identification and impeccable assessment and treatment of pain and other problems, physical, psychosocial and spiritual. (World Health Organisation, 2016)

pallor: [pal-lor]
An unnatural paleness of the skin.

palpation: [pal-pay-shun]
Physical examination whereby the examiner manually examines the body.

palsy: [paul-sy]
A weakness or paralysis of part of the body.

pancoast's tumour:
A tumour located at the highest point of the lung, which causes pain in the arm, wasting and weakening of the arm due to neurological involvement.

pancreas: [pan-kree-as]
A gland which is situated behind the stomach. The pancreas secretes enzymes which help digest food. It also secretes insulin which regulates the amount of sugar in the blood.

pancreatic carcinoma: [pan-kree-at-ik car-sin-oh-ma]
A malignant neoplastic disease of the pancreas. Common symptoms are anorexia, flatulence, weakness, weight loss, epigastric or back pain and jaundice.

pap test: (papanicolaou test)
A simple test which can detect pre-cancerous changes in the cervix. Cells are scraped from the surface of the cervix, smeared on a slide and examined under the microscope.

paraplegia: [para-plee-jia]
Paralysis of the legs, and in some cases, the lower part of the body due to a lesion in the spinal cord.

parenteral: [pah-ren-ter-al]
Outside the digestive system. E.g. drugs administered parenterally may be given by injection, subcutaneously, intravenously or intramuscularly.

pathogen: [path-o-gen]
Disease producing agent or microorganism.

pathology:
The study of the causes, nature and effects of disease.

PEG (percutaneous endoscopic gastronomy): [per-kew-tane-ious en-doh-scop-ic gas-tros-tome-ee]
An artificial opening created through the abdominal wall into the stomach, through which a tube is inserted. Sometimes used for feeding when the patient is unable to swallow due to head or neck cancer. Also used for the purpose of discharging vomit in the case of a bowel obstruction (venting PEG). The PEG may be clamped at times to allow the patient to gain some sustenance from swallowed food.

pelvic examination: [pel-vik examination]
A physical examination of the organs of the pelvis by palpation through the vagina and/or rectum.

perinatal: [perri-nate-al]
A term pertaining to the period shortly before and after birth. (includes the pre and postnatal periods.)

perinatal AIDS:
AIDS acquired by infants from their mother during pregnancy, delivery or by ingestion of contaminated breast milk.

perinatal death:
Refers to the death of the foetus weighing 400 grams or more, from 20 weeks gestation to 28 days of age.

peripheral neuropathy: [per-if-er-al nu-rop-a-thee]
A disorder characterised by altered sensation or motor function of the peripheral nervous system.

peristalsis: [pe-ri-stal-sis]
The rhythmic wave like contraction and relaxation of the smooth muscles of the oesophagus and intestines, by which contents are forced through the digestive tract.

peritoneum: [per-i-ton-eum]
An extensive membrane covering the entire internal surface of the abdominal wall and enveloping the intestines.

pharmaceutical: [fahr-muh-sue-tik-al]
In relation to drugs.

pharmacology: [fahr-muh-kol-ogee]
The science of the preparation, nature and effects of drugs on the body.

photodynamic therapy:
A treatment that uses special drugs, called photosensitizing agents, along with light to kill cancer cells. The drugs only work after they have been activated or 'turned on' by certain kinds of light.

physician:
A doctor who practices medicine not surgery. Physicians often specialise in particular body system. E.g. a neurologist specialises in the nervous system, or a gastroenterologist specialises in the gastrointestinal system.

placebo: [pla-see-boh]
An inactive substance, which resembles medicine, given instead of a drug. A placebo may be used during controlled drug trials and compared with the effect of the drug under examination.

plasma: [plaz-ma]
Colourless, watery fluid in which blood cells and platelets are suspended.

platelet: [plate-let]
Small cells in the blood which are essential for coagulation.

pleural effusion: [plur-al eff-u-shun]
An abnormal collection of fluid in the chest cavity outside the lungs. It occurs most commonly with malignancies of the bronchus, breast, lymphoma, ovary and mesothelioma (tumour of the pleura).

pneumonectomy: [nu-mon-ek-toh-mee]
The surgical removal of all or part of a lung.

pneumonia: [nu-mone-ia]
Acute inflammation of the lung.

polyp: [pol-ip]
A small growth extending on a stalk from an epithelial surface.

polyposis coli: [pol-ip-osis kole-eye]
A condition of the colon in which there is an inherited tendency to develop polyps and an increased risk of malignant transformation.

postnatal:
Occurring after the birth of an infant.

pre-cancerous: [pre-kan-sir-us]
Changes in the structure and function of tissues that may precede cancer.

premature:
Occurring before the expected time.

pressure sores:
An ulcerated area of skin caused by irritation or continuous pressure on part of the body. Also referred to as bedsores or decubitus ulcers.

prevalence:
Total number of cases of a particular disease in existence at a given time.

primary tumour:
Malignant growth at its site of origin.

prognosis: [pro-no-sis]
The prediction of the duration and outcome of the disease.

prophylactic: [proff-ill-ak-tik]
A substance (drug) used to prevent a disease or condition from developing.

prophylaxis: [proff-ill-ax-is]
The measures taken to prevent a disease.

prostate: [pross-tate]
The gland which is located at the junction of the bladder and the urethra in a man. It produces ejaculation fluid which forms part of the semen. The prostate may become enlarged in elderly men.

prostatic cancer: [pross-tat-ik kan-ser]
Cancer of the prostate.

prosthesis: [pross-thesis]
An artificial substitute for parts of the body, for functional and/or cosmetic reasons (e.g. breast, artificial limbs, pacemaker, dentures).

protocol: [pro-toh-kol]
A formalised plan for disease treatment.

pruritus: [pru-rite-us]
Itching or irritation of the skin prompting an urge to scratch. Can occur with lymphoma, liver disorders with jaundice, allergic inflammation and infection. Emotional distress may also be significant in the development of pruritus.

psychogenic: [sigh-ko-jen-ik]
A disorder which has a psychological origin as opposed to an organic basis.

psychopathology: [sigh-ko-pah-thol-o-jee)
The study of the causes, processes and manifestations of mental disorders. Also describes the behavioural manifestations of mental disorder.

psychosis: [sigh-ko-sis]
A serious mental disorder organic or emotional origin, characterised by extreme disturbance of personality, impaired perception, thinking, affect and personal orientation. The individual loses touch with reality and is severely impaired in or incapable of normal activities.

psychotropic drugs: [sigh-ko-trope-ik drugs]
Any of a large range of drugs used to modify and improve mental functioning and activity, behaviour or experience of a patient.

pubis:
The area above the external genital organs.

pulmonary: [pull-mon-rr]
Pertains to or affecting the lungs.

pyrexia: [py-rex-e-a]
High body temperature, fever.

R

rad: (radiation absorbed dose)
The basic unit of the absorbed dose of radiation.
The term is used in radiotherapy. (See **Gray**)

radiation oncologist *(see radiotherapist)*

radical surgery:
Surgical removal of a tumour plus tissue around the operative site, including muscle, lymph nodes, fat and adjacent tissues. Extensive surgery aimed to cure the disease.

radiographer: [ray-di-og-raffer]
Technician trained to take X-ray or gamma ray pictures for the diagnosis of certain diseases.

radiologist:
A physician specialising in the use of X-rays (including radionuclides), ionising radiation, Magnetic Resonance Imaging or ultrasound in the diagnosis or treatment of disease.

radionuclides: [ray-di-o-new-clydes]
A radionuclide (radioactive nuclide, radioisotope or radioactive isotope) is an atom that has excess nuclear energy.

radioresistant:
Refers to a tumour which does not respond favourable to radiotherapy.

radiotherapist: [ray-di-o-ther-a-pist]
A doctor who uses ionizing radiation (such as megavoltage X-rays or radionuclides) in the treatment of cancer. Also known as a radiation oncologist.

radiotherapy: [ray-di-o-ther-a-pee]
Treatment where X-rays or gamma rays are used to inhibit rapidly growing cells. Radiation may be directed at a tumour externally or a radioactive source may be inserted into the tumour and the surrounding tissue. Radiotherapy is particularly useful in the relief of pain from bone metastases, headache from intracranial tumours and pain from pelvic tumours. Palliative radiotherapy is usually able to be delivered with fewer doses than radiotherapy given with curative intent.

rectum: [rek-tum]
The lower end of the large intestine, ending in the anal canal.

reflux:
The abnormal return or backward flow of fluid, such as with gastro-oesophageal reflux.

regional involvement:
The spread of a cancerous growth from its original site to closely connected areas.

relapse:
The return of a disease after an interval of improvement or remission.

remission:
The disappearance or decrease of disease symptoms for a time. Complete remission refers to the absence of active disease.

renal: [ree-nal]
Relating to the kidneys.

renal cancer:
Cancer of the kidneys.

resection: [re-section]
Surgical removal of all or part of an organ. (Resection may be complete or partial.)

respiratory system: [re-spi-rah-tory system]
The group of organs and structures that contribute to breathing: the nose, mouth, trachea, bronchial tubes and lungs.

retina:
A layered nervous tissue membrane at the back of the eye, continuous with the optic nerve, that is light sensitive and able to receive and transmit images of external objects through the optic nerve to the brain.

retinitis:
Inflammation of the retina.

retinoblastoma: [ret-i-no-blass-to-mah]
A malignant tumour of nerve cells of the retina.

retroperitoneal: [ret-roh-per-i-toh-neal]
Refers to the structures situated between the posterior abdominal wall and the posterior layer of the peritoneum (nerves, arteries, veins, lymph nodes, and parts of the bowel).

rhabdomyosarcoma: [rab-doh-my-oh-sar-ko-mah]
A malignant growth or striated or skeletal muscle. The tumour grows rapidly and tends to metastasise early.

robotic surgery:
A form of robot-assisted surgery that allows doctors to perform many types of complex procedures with more precision, flexibility and control than is possible with conventional techniques. This form of surgery is becoming more common for prostate cancer surgery.

S

sacrum: [say-krum]
Triangular wedge-shaped bone, situated between the lowest lumbar vertebra and the coccyx. It is located between the back of the hip bones.

sarcoma: [sar-ko-ma]
A malignant tumour of the soft tissue arising in muscle, cartilage, bone or the lymphatic system.

scan:
A two-dimensional image of deep tissues produced by a machine using gamma radiation or sound waves. Scans are valuable in diagnosing and determining the spread of cancer.

secondary tumour:
A tumour which develops in the body distant from the primary tumour sue to the spread of cancer cells.

seizure: [see-zure]
Sudden and violent involuntary contractions of a group of muscles. Also known as a convulsion or fit.

septicaemia: [sep-ti-see-mee-a]
A systemic blood infection which may originate from an infection in any part of the body.

serum: (seer-um)
The clear fluid portion of blood remaining when the blood cells, platelets and clotting substances (fibrinogen) are removed. If fibrinogen is not removed the clear fluid is called plasma.

shunt:
A diversion of the flow of a body fluid from one cavity or vessel to another. A tube or device may be implanted into the body to facilitate the redirection of the body fluid.

SIDS: (Sudden Infant Death Syndrome)
The unexpected and sudden death of an apparently normal healthy infant during sleep, with no physical evidence of disease. It is the most common cause of death of infants between 2 weeks and 1 year.

sigmoid: [sig-moid]
The S shaped portion of the colon or sigmoid colon.

sigmoidectomy: [sig-moid-ek-toh-mee]
The surgical excision of part of the sigmoid colon, most commonly performed to remove a cancerous tumour.

skin cancer:
A skin tumour caused by ionising radiation, genetic defects, chemical carcinogens or by over exposure to the sun or other ultraviolet light. Skin cancer is the most common form of cancer in Australia. (See **basal cell carcinoma, squamous cell carcinoma, melanoma**.)

small cell carcinoma:
A malignant tumour usually of the lung. One third of all malignant tumours of the lung are of this type, and of all lung cancers it is the type most likely to respond to chemotherapy.

small intestine:
The section of the gastro-intestinal tract located between the stomach and the colon. It is also referred to as the small bowel.

solar keratosis: [soh-lar ker-a-toh-sis]
A flattened reddened scaly area which appears on skin exposed to sunlight. A solar keratosis is not skin cancer, but an indication that the patient may be prone to skin cancer.

spleen:
An organ situated in the upper part of the abdomen on the left side. Functions of the spleen include the manufacture of white blood cells and the breakdown of red blood cells.

splenomegaly: [sple-no-meg-a-lee]
Enlargement of the spleen.

spurious diarrhoea: [spure-ee-is dye-uh-rea] (see **faecal impaction**)

sputum cytology test: [spu-tum sight-ology test]
A test which studies cells in sputum from the lungs and air passages.

squamous cell carcinoma: [squay-mus cell kar-si-no-ma]
A malignant tumour originating in squamous (scaly) epithelium (surface layer of cells), May occur in the lungs, skin, anus, cervix, nose and bladder.

stem cells:
Immature blood cells found in bone marrow and blood, with the special ability to mature into all types of blood cells. Certain types of cancer can be treated and in some cases cured with a stem cell transplant.

steroids: [steer-oids]
A large number of hormonal substances including oestrogens, androgens, progesterone and corticosteroids. They may occur naturally or may be synthesised. They are useful in relieving pain due to swelling associated with a cancer. (See **pharmaceutical section**)

stoma: [stow-ma]
A surgically created opening in the skin usually described by the anatomical name of the opening. (e.g. tracheostomy, colostomy or ileostomy). (See **ostomy**)

stomach cancer: (See **gastric carcinoma**)

stomal therapist: [stow-mal therapist]
A professional trained in the care of stomas.

stridor:
A peculiar harsh or high-pitched sound indicating some obstruction to the breathing.

subcutaneous: [sub-ku-tane-eus]
Beneath the skin.

subcutaneous injection:
Injection into the tissue immediately beneath the skin, for the delivery of a single dose of medication, or continuous infusion.

Sudden Infant Death Syndrome: (See **SIDS**)

suppository:
A dissolvable bullet shaped vehicle for medication which is inserted into the rectum or vagina.

suprapubic:
Above the pubis.

survival rates:
Refers to the study of a group of people with the same disease, tracing how many are still alive after a given time from the time of diagnosis. The rate refers to the proportion or percentage of the group surviving.

symptomatic treatment:
Palliative treatment seeking to relieve a patient's symptoms rather than cure the disease.

syringe driver:
A device which allows delivery of continuous subcutaneous medication for symptom control, when the oral route is unsatisfactory. The aim is to provide optimum patient comfort, mobility and independence while receiving medication.

T

tachypnoea: [tak-ip-nee-ah]
An abnormally rapid rate of breathing.

targeted cancer therapies:
Drugs or other substances that block the growth and spread of cancer by interfering with specific molecules ('molecular targets') that are involved in the growth, progression, and spread of cancer.

terminal:
Expectation that a patient's survival can be measured by days, weeks or months.

terminal restlessness: (See **agitation**)

testicular cancer: [tes-tik-u-lar cancer]
A malignant tumour of the testes, occurring most frequently in men between 20-35 years of age. The most common cancers of the testis are seminomas (70%) and teratomas (25-30%).

therapy: [ther-a-pee]
Treatment which may be:
a) Specific – expected to influence favourably the course of the disease.
b) Symptomatic – relieving the symptoms without altering the course of the disease.

thoracic: [thor-ass-ik]
Relating to or affecting the chest.

thoracic spine: [thor-ass-ik spine]
The section of the backbone between the neck and the lower back.

thrombocytopenia: [throm-boh-sigh-toh-pee-nia]
A reduced number of blood platelets resulting in the blood taking longer to clot. This may be the result of chemotherapy or bone marrow being replaced by cancerous cells. Spontaneous bleeding may occur.

thrombosis: [throm-bo-sis]
The formation of a blood clot within a blood vessel.

thrush: (See **candida**)

tomography: [toh-mog-ra-fee] (See **CAT scan**)

toxicity: [tok-sis-i-tee]
The degree of virulence of a drug or poison. (e.g. the drugs used in chemotherapy can have undesirable side effects due to their level of toxicity).

trachea: [tra-kee-uh]
The windpipe. It extends from the lower part of the larynx to the beginning of the bronchi.

tracheostomy: [trak-ee-os-toh-mee]
The creation of a stoma (artificial opening) into the trachea.

transfusion:
The introduction of whole blood or a blood component into a vein.

tumour:
An abnormal swelling. A tumour can either be benign or malignant.
Also called a neoplasm.

U

ulcer:
Erosion of the skin or mucous membrane.
e.g. mouth ulcers following chemotherapy, or pressure sores resulting
from lying immobile for extended periods.

ultrasound:
The use of high frequency soundwaves to examine the interior organs
of the body. Ultrasonic waves may be used in the treatment of soft
tissue pain.

undifferentiated cells:
Immature cells which are not developed sufficiently to conduct their
specified function.

uraemia: [u-ree-mi-a]
A condition of high blood urea. There is muscle weakness and
increasing drowsiness produced by renal failure.

urethra: [u-ree-thra]
The passage from the bladder to allow the passing of urine.

urinary tract:
The system of body parts which leads urine from the kidneys to the
exterior of the body.

urodome: [u-ro-dome]
An open-ended condom to which a urinary drainage bag is attached
(an external catheter).

urologist: [u-rol-o-gist]
A doctor specialising in diseases of the urinary tract.

uterine cancer:
Any malignancy of the uterus. It may be cervical cancer affecting the
cervix or endometrial cancer affecting the lining of the body of the
uterus.

uterus:
A triangular shaped, hollow, muscular organ in the female pelvis. It is situated in the pelvic cavity between the bladder and the rectum. Its function is to provide nourishment and protection for the foetus during pregnancy, and expulsion at the time of birth.

V

vagina:
The lower part of the female reproductive system. A muscular canal which leads from the cervix of the uterus to the vulva.

vaginal thrush:
Infection of the vagina caused by a microscopic yeast-like fungal organism, candida albicans, sometimes resulting in itching and a weeping white discharge. (See *candida*)

vascular: [vass-kew-lar]
Referring to or consisting of blood vessels.

ventilator:
A machine which inflates lungs in a rhythmical manner through an endotracheal or tracheostomy tube. A respirator.

vertebra: [ver-te-bra]
The 33 irregular shaped bones which together from the spinal column. There are: 7 cervical, 12 thoracic, 5 lumbar, 5 sacral (sacrum) and 4 coccygeal (coccyx) vertebra.

vomit:
Contents of the stomach ejected through the month.
a) Bilious vomit – vomit and bile
b) Coffee-ground – contains small quantities of blood and has the appearance of ground coffee
c) Faecal – vomit and faeces.

vulva: [vul-va]
The external female genital organs.

W

white blood cell:
Known as a leucocyte. The three types of mature white blood cells are:
1. Granulocytes (neutrophils and eosinophils).
2. Lymphocytes.
3. Monocytes

Granulocytes and monocytes are produced in the bone marrow, while lymphocytes are produced in the lymph nodes. White blood cells act to defend the body against infection.

wilms' tumour:
A rare but highly malignant tumour of the kidney (affecting children under 8 years).
Known also as nephroblastoma.

X

xerostomia: [zero-sto-mia]
A dryness of the mouth due to lack of normal salivary secretion.

x-rays:
Short length electromagnetic waves used to penetrate tissue to form an image of the internal structure of the body on photographic film or screen. They are used to aid diagnosis, and treat disease.

ABBREVIATIONS IN PALLIATIVE CARE

#	FRACTURE
AC	Before Meals
AIDS	Acquired Immune Defiency Syndrome
BCC	Basal Cell Carcinoma
BD	Twice Daily
CAT (CT)	Computerised Axial Tomography Scan
CBE	Complete Blood Examination
CCF	Congestive Cardiac Failure
CNS	Central Nervous System
COAD	Chronic Obstructive Airways Disease
COPD	Chronic Obstructive Pulmonary Disease
CSCI (or SCI)	(Continuous) Subcutaneous Infusion
CVA	Cerebro-vascular Accident
DVT	Deep Vein Thrombosis
FBE	Full Blood Examination
FNA	Fine Needle Aspirate (see Cytology)
GIT	Gastro-intestinal Tract
Gy	Gray
HDC	Hypodermoclysis
HIV	Human Immunodeficiency Virus
HSV	Herpes Simplex Virus
IDC	Indwelling (Urinary) Catheter
IV	Intravenous
IVT	Intravenous Therapy
MRI	Magnetic Resonance Imaging
M/T	Mouth Toilet
NAD	No Abnormality Detected
NIDDM	Non-insulin Dependent Dabetes Mellitus
NSAID	Non-steroidal Anti-inflammatory Drugs
PAC	Pressure Area Care
PC	After Meals
PR	Per Rectum
PRN	Pro re nata or as the situation arises
QID	Four Times Daily
R/T	Radiotherapy
SCC	Squamous Cell Carcinoma
SOB	Short Of Breath
Stat	At Once
TDS	Three Times Daily
TENS	Transcutaneous Electrical Nerve Stimulation

MEDICATIONS COMMONLY USED FOR SYMPTOM MANAGEMENT

	GENERIC DRUG NAME	BRAND NAME(S)
Agitation	Clonazepam	Rivotril, Paxam
	Diazepam	Valium, Antenex, Ducene
	Midazolam	Hypnovel
Anti-convulsant	Levetiracetam	Keppra
	Sodium Valproate	Epilim
	Diazepam	Valium
	Lorazepam	Ativan
Anti-inflammatories	Prednisone	Sone, Predsone, Panafcort
	Dexamethasone	Decadron, Dexasone, Diodex, Hexadrol, Maxidex
Non-steroidal anti-inflammatories	Aspirin	Aspro Clear, Cartia
	Celecoxib	Celebrex
	Diclofenac	Cataflam, Voltaren-XR
	Ibuprofen	Motrin, Advil
Anti-psychotic *(See Psychosis)*		
Anxiety	Midazolam	Hypnovel
	Lorazepam	Ativan
	Alprazolam	Xanax, Kalma
	Oxazepam	Serepax, Alepam, Murelax
Ascites	Furosemide	Lasix, Uremide, Urex
	Spironolactone	Aldactone, Spiractin
Blood Clotting	Warfarin	Marevan, Coumadin
	Dabigatran etexilate	Pradaxa
	Rivaroxaban	Xarelto
	Apixaban	Eliquis
Confusion	Diazepam	Valium, Antenex, Ducene
	Haloperidol	Serenace
	Midazolam	Hypnovel
Cough	Morphine	Ordine
	Lignocaine	Xylocaine
	Linctus Gee	Actacode
	Codeine Linctus (QLD only)	
Death rattle	Atropine	Lomotil
	Hyoscine hydrobromide	Buscopan
	Glycopyrrolate	Hospira

Delayed gastric emptying	Metoclopramide	Maxolon, Pramin
	Domperidone	Motilium
Depression	Amitriptyline	Endep, Tyrptanol
	Citalopram	Celepram
	Dothiepin	Prothiaden, Dothep
	Escitalopram	Lexapro
	Duloxetine	Cymbalta
	Fluoxetine	Prozac, Lovan,
	Mirtazapine	Avanza
	Nortriptyline	Allegron
	Paroxetine	Zactin
	Sertraline	Aropax
	Venlafaxine	Zoloft, Efexor-XR
Diarrhoea	Loperamide	Gastrex, Imodium
Dyspnoea	Dexamethasone	Decadron, Dexasone, Diodex, Hexadrol, Maxidex
	Diazepam	Valium, Antenex, Ducene
	Lignocaine	Xylocaine
	Prednisone	Sone, Predsone, Panafcort
	Midazolam	Hypnovel
	Salbutamol	Sandoz
	Morphine (and other opioids) Ordine	
Hypercalcaemia	Zoledronic acid	Zometa
	Pamidronate sodium	Aredia
Insomnia	Temazepam	Temaze, Euhypnos, Normison
	Nitrazepam	Mogadon, Alodorm
Intestinal Obstruction	Hyoscine-N-butyl bromide	Buscopan
	Serenace	Haloperidol
	Sandostatin	Octreotide
Laxative	Bisacodyl	Petrus
	Danthron	
	Poloxamer	
	Docusate	Coloxyl
	Docusate sodium	Hypnovel
	Lactulose	Actilix, Duphalac
	Sodium citrate	Microlax
	Sorbitol	Micolette, Movicol
	Sennosides	Senokot

Nausea	Cyclizine	Valoid
	Domperidone	Motilium
	Haloperidol	Serenace
	Metoclopramide	Maxolon, Pramin
	Prochlorperazine	Stemetil
	Ondansetron	Zofran, Ondaz
	Tropisetron	Navoban
Haemorrhage	Tranexamic acid	Cyklokapron
Oedema	Spironolactone	Aldactone, Spiractin
Oral Care	Miconazole	Daktarin
	Nystatin	Nilstat
Psychosis	Haloperidol	Serenace
	Levomepromazine (methotrimeprazine)	Nozinan, Levoprome
	Olanzapine	Zyprexa
	Quetiapine	Seroquel
	Risperidone	Riserdal
Terminal restlessness	Midazolam	Hypnovel
	Levomepromazine	Nozinan
Ulcers & Reflux	Ranitidine	Zantac
Wound Care	Metronidazole	Rozex

MEDICATIONS COMMONLY USED FOR PAIN MANAGEMENT

ORAL	GENERIC DRUG NAME	BRAND NAME(S)
Opioid induced sedation or cognitive failure	Methylphenidate	Ritalin, Concerta
Opioid sensitive pain	Morphine Kapanol	Ordine, MS Contin
	Oxycodone	Endone Proladone
	Hydromorphone	Dilaudid
	Tramadol	Zaldiar
	Fentanyl	Sandoz
	Methadone	Physeptone, Dolophine, Methadose
	Buprenorphine	Subutex
Non-opioid sensitive pain		
Anti-convulsant	Gabapentin	Gabapentin Sandoz
	Pregabalin	Lyrica
	Carbamazepine	Tegretol, Teril
	Sodium Valproate	Epilim, Valpro
Antidepressants	Amitriptyline	Endep, Tryptanol
	Nortriptyline	Pamelor
	Dothiepin	Prothiaden, Dothep
Anti-inflammatories	Aspirin	Aspro Clear, Cartia
	Naproxen	Naprosyn
	Diclofenec	Voltaren
	Ketorolac	Toradol
Corticosteroid	Dexamethasone	Dexamethasone
Muscle relaxants	Diazepam	Valium, Antenex,
	Clonazepam	Rivotril, Paxam
	Baclofen	Lioresal, Clofen

PARENTERAL	GENERIC DRUG NAME	BRAND NAMES (S)
NMDA Receptor Antagonist	Ketamine	Ketalar
	Methadone	Catapres
Alpha 2 Agonist	Clonidine	Apo

PREFIXES AND SUFFIXES

a-, an-	not, without
acr-	extremely, peak
ad-	towards
adeno-	gland
adip-	fat
-aemia	blood
aer-	air
-aesthesia	sensation
-algia	pain
amyl-	starch
ana-	up
andr-	male
angi-	(blood) vessel
ante-	before, infront
anti-	against
apo-	away, from
arthr-	joint
-asis	state of
aut-	self
bi-, bis-	two
bil-	bile
bio	life
blast-	bud
blephar-	eyelid
brachi-	arm
bracy-	short
brady-	slow
bronch-	windpipe
calc-	chalk
carcin-	cancer
card-	heart
carp-	wrist
cata-, kata-	down, negative
cav-	hollow
-cele	swelling
cent-	hundred
-centesis	piercing
cerphal-	head
cerebr-	brain
cervic-	neck
cheil-, chil-,	lip
cheir-, chir-	hand
chol-	bile
chondr-	cartilage
chrom-	colour
-cide	killing
cine-, kine-	motion
-cle	small
co-, col-, com-, con-	together with
colp-	vagina
contra-	against, counter
cortic-	bark, rind
cost-	rib
cox-	hip
crani-	skull
cryo-	cold
crypt-	hidden, concealed
cysan-	blue
cyst-	bladder
cyt-	cell
-cyte	cell
dactyl-	finger
de-	down, from
dec-	ten
demi-	half
dent-	tooth
derm-	skin
-desis	binding
dextr-	right
di-, diplo-	two, double
dia-	through
dis-	apart, away from
dors-	back
dys-	difficult, abnormal
ect-	outside
-ectasis	stretching
-ectomy	cutting out
em-, en-, end-, ent-	in, inside, without
enter-	intestine
epi-	upon, over
erythr-	red
eu-	good, normal
ex-, exo-	out of
extra-	outside

faci-	face	-malacia	softening
-facient	making	mamm-	breast
flav-	yellow	mast-	breast
galact-	milk	medi	middle
gastr-	stomach	megal-	large
-genic	producing	melan-	black
ger-	old age	meso-	middle
gloss-	tongue	meta-	after
glyc-	sweet	metr-	uterus
gnath-	jaw	micr-	small
-gram	recorded	milli-	thousand
-graph	tracing	mono-	single
gynae-	female	-morph	form
haem-	blood	muco-	mucus
hemi	half	multi-	many
hepat-	liver	myc-	fungus
hex-	six	myel-	marrow
hist-	tissue, web	myo-	muscle
hom-	same, like	narc-	numb
hydr-	water	naso-	nose
hyper-	above	necr-	corpse
hypno-	sleep	neo-	new
hypo-	below	nephr-	kidney
hyster-	womb	neur-	nerve
-ia, -iasis	state, condition	ocul-	eye
idi-	peculiar, distinct	odont-	tooth
infra-	below	-odynia	pain
inter-	between	-oid	like
intra-	within	oligo-	few
intro-	inwards	Oology	study
iso-	equal	-oma	tumour
-it is	inflammation of	onco-	mass
kary-	nut, nucleus	onych-	nail
kerat-	horn, cornea	oo-	egg
-kinesis,	motion	ophthalm-	eye
-kinetic		-opsy	looking
lact-	milk	or-	mouth
laryng-	windpipe	otchid-	testis
later-	side	orth-	straight
leuc-, leuk-	white	os-	mouth
-lith	stone	os-, oste-	bone
-lysis	destruction	-osis	pathological state
macr-	large	-ostomy	opening
mal-	bad, abnormal	ot-	ear

-otomy	cutting	-rrhoea	discharge
ovi-	egg	-rrhapy	repair
pachy-	thick	rub-	red
paed-	child	salping-	(uterine) tube
pan-	all	sarc-	flesh
para-	beside, beyond	sclero-	hard
path-	suffering, disease	-scope	viewing instrument
-pathy	disease	-scopy	looking
-penia	lack	semi-	half
pent-	five	sept-	seven
per-	through	-sonic	sound
peri-	around	sphygm-	pulse
-pexy	fixing	splen-	spleen
-phagia	swallowing	spondy-	vertebra
pharmac-	drug	steat-	fat
-phasia	speech	sub-	below
phleb-	vein	super-, supra-	above
-phobia	irrational fear	syn-	with
phon-	sound	tachy-	quick
photo-	light	tars-	eyelid, instep
phren-	diaphragm, mind	-taxia, taxis	arrangement, order
-phylaxis	prevention, protection	tetra-	four
physi-	form, nature	therm-	heat
-plegia	paralysis	thorac-	chest
pneum-	lung	thromb-	clot
pod-	foot	-tome	cutting instrument
-poiesis	formation	toxic-	poison
poly-	many	trans-	through, across
post-	after	tri-	three
prae-, pre-, pro-	before, in front	trich,	hair
proct-	anus	troph-	nourishment
pseud-	false	-tropic	turning
psych-	mind	tympano-	middle ear
pyo-	pus, matter	ultra-	beyond
pyr-	fire, fever	uni-	one
quadr-	four	uri-	urine
quint-	five	-uria	urine
radi-	ray	vas-	vessel
re-	back, again	xanth-	yellow
ren-	kidney	xero-	dry
retro-	backwards	zoo-	animal
rhin-	nose		

REFERENCES

Anderson, K., Anderson, L. and Glanze, W. (1998). *Mosby's medical, nursing, & allied health dictionary*. St. Louis: Mosby.

American Cancer Society, *Information and Resources for Cancer: Breast, Colon, Lung, Prostate, Skin*. (2016). *cancer.org*. http://www.cancer.org/index

Ashfield, J. and Lockyer-Scrutton, P. (1998). *Dictionary of medical and pharmaceutical terms for bereavement and palliative care counsellors*. North Adelaide, S. Aust.: Calvary Hospital Adelaide.

Burr, G. (1991). *Baillière's Australian nurses' dictionary*. Sydney: Baillière Tindall.
Diagnostic and Statistical Manual of Mental Disorders. (2013) (5th ed.). London.

Kaye, P. (1990). *Notes on symptom control in hospice & palliative care*. Essex, Conn., USA: Hospice Education Institute.
Oxford Dictionaries - Dictionary, Thesaurus, & Grammar. (2016). *Oxford Dictionaries | English*. Retrieved 26 October 2016, from https://en.oxforddictionaries.com/

MacLeod, R., Vella-Brincat, J., & Macleod, A. (2014). *The palliative care handbook: Guidelines for clinical management and symptom control*. Sydney Australia: Hammond Press.

Medicines. (2016). *npsmedicinewise*. http://www.nps.org.au/medicines

Palliative Drugs. (2016). *palliativedrugs.com*. http://www.palliativedrugs.com/

Potter, D. (1983). *Assessment*. Springhouse, Pa.: Intermed Communications.

Scottish Palliative Care Guidelines - Home. (2016). *palliativecareguidelines.scot.nhs.uk*. http://www.palliativecareguidelines.scot.nhs.uk/

Solzhenitsyn, A. (1973). *The cancer ward*. New York: Dell.

Urdang, L. and Swallow, H. (1983). *Mosby's medical & nursing dictionary*. St. Louis: C.V. Mosby Co.

Wilkes, G. & Krebs, W. (2016). *Oxford Dictionaries - Dictionary, Thesaurus, & Grammar. Oxford Dictionaries | English*. https://en.oxforddictionaries.com/

WHO | WHO Definition of Palliative Care. (2016). *Who.int*. http://www.who.int/cancer/palliative/definition/en/

USEFUL RESOURCES

The Palliative Care Bridge resource website: has an excellent video series and other resources: www.palliativecarebridge.com.au

Palliative Care Guidelines Plus http://www.Book.pallcare.info/

www.ingramcontent.com/pod-product-compliance
Lightning Source LLC
Chambersburg PA
CBHW070909210326
41521CB00010B/2113